Andrea Benevides Leite

Risk Factors for NASH in Cryptogenic Cirrhosis

Andrea Benevides Leite

Risk Factors for NASH in Cryptogenic Cirrhosis

A prevalence study in southern Brazil

ScienciaScripts

Imprint

Any brand names and product names mentioned in this book are subject to trademark, brand or patent protection and are trademarks or registered trademarks of their respective holders. The use of brand names, product names, common names, trade names, product descriptions etc. even without a particular marking in this work is in no way to be construed to mean that such names may be regarded as unrestricted in respect of trademark and brand protection legislation and could thus be used by anyone.

Cover image: www.ingimage.com

This book is a translation from the original published under ISBN 978-613-9-69166-1.

Publisher:
Sciencia Scripts
is a trademark of
Dodo Books Indian Ocean Ltd. and OmniScriptum S.R.L publishing group

120 High Road, East Finchley, London, N2 9ED, United Kingdom
Str. Armeneasca 28/1, office 1, Chisinau MD-2012, Republic of Moldova, Europe
Printed at: see last page
ISBN: 978-620-6-46010-7

I dedicate this work to my parents, Vera and
Eduardo, inexhaustible sources of love and support,
and to my son Arthur, God's light in my life.

ACKNOWLEDGMENTS

To God, who allowed me to take this journey.

To Dr. Angelo Mattos - with whom I have had the great opportunity to live and whom I have come to admire for his professional and human qualities - for the kindness with which he welcomed me into his service, for his support in times of difficulty, and for the patience and skill with which he guided me during my Master's degree.

To my friend Dr. Sérgio Pessoa, an example of a doctor, to whom I owe all the opportunities in Gastroenterology, for his dedication to teaching during my years of Residency and for always encouraging me to do research.

To Dr. Gabriela Coral, Dr. Sandro Evaldt and everyone who contributed in any way to the development of this work.

To my friend Luciani Spencer, secretary of the Graduate Program at UFCSPA, for her kindness and constant willingness to help.

To the invaluable friends I met in Porto Alegre - RS, who made my stay away from home enjoyable.

To the patients, the subjects of this research.

SUMMARY

Cryptogenic cirrhosis represents the final stage of some occult chronic liver diseases, with non-alcoholic steatohepatitis (NASH) being one of the main underlying diseases responsible for these cases. Some studies have looked for an association between cryptogenic cirrhosis and NASH by comparing the "metabolic profile" of the two groups, emphasizing diabetes mellitus and obesity. The aim of this study was to determine the prevalence of risk factors for NASH in patients with cryptogenic cirrhosis in Porto Alegre, in the southern region of Brazil, in order to establish a possible causal relationship. It was prepared and presented as a dissertation to the Postgraduate Course in Hepatology at the Federal University of Health Sciences of Porto Alegre to obtain a Master's degree in Hepatology, under the supervision of Professor Angelo Alves de Mattos and co-supervision of Professor Gabriela Perdomo Coral. The literature review was carried out in the light of existing knowledge up to 2011.

The study was carried out at ISCMPA's Gastroenterology Department between 2008 and 2010, involving 47 patients with cryptogenic cirrhosis, 47 with NASH and 196 with cirrhosis caused by HCV and/or alcohol, with assessment of the following variables: glycemia, body mass index, total cholesterol, HDL and triglycerides, as well as age, gender and Child-Pugh score.

In patients with cryptogenic cirrhosis, the prevalence of altered fasting glucose levels / DM was 68.2%; obesity, 27.5%; hypercholesterolemia, 27.9%; low HDL levels, 58.1%, 81% in women and 36.4% in men; and hypertriglyceridemia, 16.3%. Comparison with the profile of NASH patients shows statistical similarity only between the glycemic profile (62.8%) and HDL levels in male patients (53.8%). The comparison with other cirrhotic patients shows a statistical difference between the glycemic profile (45.2%), total cholesterol (13.3%) and HDL levels in female patients (50.8%). The mean age of patients with cryptogenic cirrhosis was 52 years, while that of patients with NASH was 46.4 years, around 6 years lower, p = 0.041. The group with cryptogenic cirrhosis had 23 female and 24 male patients. Those with NASH were predominantly female (68.1%) and those with cirrhosis caused by alcohol and/or HCV were predominantly male (64.8%), with no statistical difference between either group.

We conclude that, in assessing the possible etiological relationship between NASH and cryptogenic cirrhosis, the results of this study only allow us to make an inference, given the concordance of the glycemic profile and the difference in mean age, which suggests a time needed for the eventual progression of the disease. It is not possible to establish a causal relationship with the results obtained, and a prospective study with a larger number of patients would be interesting.

Keywords: Cryptogenic cirrhosis, NASH, metabolic syndrome.

TABLE OF CONTENTS

CHAPTER 1 - INTRODUCTION

Cirrhosis is a clinical condition that represents the final stage common to several chronic liver diseases and is one of the main causes of mortality worldwide. It is characterized by lobular and vascular architectural disorganization of the liver, with the formation of nodules, resulting from the diffuse destruction of the liver parenchyma by chronic aggression.[1]

The established hepatocellular and vascular damage leads to a series of disorders, resulting in hepatocyte insufficiency and portal hypertension.[1] The clinical picture of decompensated cirrhosis is severe, resulting in conditions that can lead to death. Patients with decompensated cirrhosis can suffer from upper gastrointestinal bleeding due to ruptured gastroesophageal varices; hepatic encephalopathy; ascites; spontaneous bacterial peritonitis ; hepatorenal syndrome; hepato-pulmonary syndrome and decreased myocardial response to stress. ,[12] In addition to these complications, there is a risk of hepatocellular carcinoma (HCC), the annual incidence of which varies between 1 and 4%.[3,4,5,6]

Cirrhosis is the main cause of indication for liver transplantation, the others being represented mainly by cases of acute liver failure, HCC and cholestatic liver diseases with intractable pruritus.[1]

In Brazil, more than a thousand liver transplants are performed every year. In 2010, 1,295 liver transplants were carried out using cadaveric donors (1,404 when adding living donors).[7] However, the difference between the number of potential recipients and the number of organs available highlights the need to control the progression of chronic liver diseases.

There are several etiologies of cirrhosis.[8] Knowing them is a fundamental step in intervening in the natural course of the disease, in order to prevent or slow down its progression. However, there are situations in which even after detailed clinical, serological and anatomopathological studies, it is not possible to clarify the underlying chronic liver disease.[9-14] In these cases, cirrhosis is called cryptogenic, cryptogenetic or idiopathic. In studies published between 1981 and 1990, we found a prevalence of 14 to 43% of cryptogenic cirrhosis in cases of chronic liver disease.[15-21] However, according to studies carried out after the discovery of the hepatitis C virus (HCV), this prevalence is below 10% (3 to 9.9%).[9,22-25]

The etiology of cryptogenic cirrhosis is not credited to a specific underlying disease, but possibly to the final stage of some hidden chronic diseases.[11] The diseases most widely accepted as possible causes are non-alcoholic steatohepatitis (NASH), silent autoimmune hepatitis, hepatitis caused by an as yet unknown virus and unreported alcoholism.[9-14]

Stephen Caldwell and colleagues,[9] in 1999, carried out a study of 70 patients diagnosed with cryptogenic cirrhosis, in which observations were made regarding risk factors for the main suspected diseases. They considered data such as the presence of type 2 diabetes mellitus (DM) and/or obesity, blood transfusion before the diagnosis of cirrhosis, and a score > 10 on the International Autoimmune Hepatitis score. They observed that the most prevalent were the presence of DM (53%) and obesity (47%), followed by FAN (anti-nuclear factor) > 1:40 (44%). The authors were able to isolate 25 patients (35.7%) with only risk factors for NASH and 19 (27.1%) with predominantly autoimmune findings. At the same time, the authors also compared the prevalence of DM and obesity in the 70 cases of cryptogenic cirrhosis with the prevalence in 39 patients with HCV cirrhosis and 33 with primary biliary cirrhosis (PBC), as well as in 50 non-cirrhotic patients with NASH. The prevalence of DM and obesity in patients with cryptogenic cirrhosis was similar to that of those with NASH (42% DM and 64% obesity), and was higher than that found in patients cirrhotic due to HCV (25% DM and 3% obesity) and CBP (15% DM and 15% obesity). In this study, the authors draw a correlation between the mean age of patients with NASH, 49 years, and that of cases with cryptogenic cirrhosis, 63 years, drawing attention to the natural history of NASH, which can progress to cirrhosis over the years.

Following the line of research into risk factors for non-alcoholic fatty liver disease (NAFLD), the following year Poonawala and collaborators[24] published a study in which they compared the prevalence of DM and obesity in 49 cases of cryptogenic cirrhosis with 98 controls matched for gender and age, with a similar Child-Pugh score, listed for liver transplantation. The underlying liver disease of the control patients included alcohol, hepatitis B virus (HBV), autoimmune hepatitis, primary sclerosing cholangitis, and others, in addition to CBP and HCV-related liver disease, increasing the representativeness of chronic liver diseases. The results obtained corroborate the study by Caldwell et al: 47% of the cases were obese versus 24% of the controls; 47% had DM versus 22% of the controls; and 23% were obese and diabetic versus 5% of the controls. The prevalence of DM among cases of cryptogenic cirrhosis was 4 times higher than the rate in the American population, and that of obesity was almost 2 times higher. The authors reinforce the hypothesis that NASH is one of the important causes of cryptogenic cirrhosis.

In 2003, a Japanese study was published[25] in which the authors assessed 404 cirrhotic patients for the prevalence of obesity and DM. A total of 40 patients (9.9% of the sample) had cryptogenic cirrhosis and these had a higher prevalence of obesity - 53% - and DM - 40% - when compared to the other cirrhotic patients (control group) who had a prevalence of 20 and 18%, respectively.

In 2008, Tellez-Avila and colleagues[26] conducted a similar study evaluating the relationship between metabolic syndrome and cryptogenic cirrhosis. In this study, the authors also compared the prevalence of obesity and DM in a group with cryptogenic cirrhosis versus a group composed of cirrhotics due to HCV, alcohol and autoimmune hepatitis (control group). The study included 134 patients with cryptogenic cirrhosis, 81 with HCV cirrhosis, 33 with alcohol cirrhosis and 20 with autoimmune hepatitis. The mean Child-Pugh score was not statistically different between the groups. DM was present in 40% of cases versus 22.4% of controls, p =0.013. As for obesity, the difference was statistically significant (16.4% vs. 8.2%) when the control group was assessed together, but there was no difference when each subgroup was assessed separately. Incidentally, the prevalence of overweight was also assessed and showed no statistical difference between the groups. In this article, the authors still study the prevalence of dyslipidemia, however, they approach hypertriglyceridemia and low HDL as a single variable. They found a prevalence of dyslipidemia in cryptogenic cirrhosis of 54% versus 6% in the control group, p <0.001, a difference that is maintained when analyzing each subgroup of the control.

In 1996, one of the first studies to correlate NASH with cryptogenic cirrhosis was carried out by evaluating the recurrence of NASH in the transplanted liver. In this article, Kim and colleagues[27] studied 7 patients who developed cirrhosis due to NASH and underwent liver transplantation. They detected the recurrence of steatosis in 5, 3 of which progressed to steatohepatitis. An eighth patient was transplanted for cryptogenic cirrhosis. In this case, the authors detected the development of moderate steatosis 4 months after transplantation, which could suggest NASH as a possible etiology of cirrhosis.

Similar to this study is the article by Sutedja et al.[28] with 37.6% development of steatosis versus 16.7% of controls, 25% of whom had NASH, and by Sanjeevi et al.[29] with 11.3% development of NASH in those transplanted for cryptogenic cirrhosis.

Mixing the two types of design - study of the clinical profile and post-transplant recurrence - Janus Ong and collaborators[30] showed recurrence of steatosis or steatohepatitis in 52% of patients transplanted for cryptogenic cirrhosis who had at least 1 post-transplant biopsy (25 out of 51 cases of cryptogenic cirrhosis transplanted). The clinical data studied allows a comparison of the 8 cases in which NASH was diagnosed with the 12 cases in which no signs of NAFLD were found: prevalence of DM - 62.5 x 8.3%; mean triglycerides (TG) - 285.9 x 117.7 mg/dL; mean body mass index (BMI) - 28.4 x 27.3 kg/m^2 .

Along the same lines, Ayata et al.[10] described in 2002 the clinical data and histopathological findings of the explant of 27 patients with cryptogenic cirrhosis who had undergone liver transplantation. They concluded that 33% of cases (9 patients) corresponded to NASH and 22% (6 patients) to autoimmune hepatitis. During post-transplant follow-up, 2 of the 9 patients diagnosed with NASH had a recurrence of the disease. The pre-transplant clinical profile was assessed and DM was found in 3 of the 9 NASH cases, in 2 of the 6 autoimmune hepatitis cases and in the only HCV case, while it was not seen in any of the other 11 cases. Obesity was found in 5 of the 9 NASH cases, in 2 of the 6 autoimmune hepatitis cases and in none of the other 12 cases.

Most of the studies cited above are American. In Europe, similar studies have also shown

NASH to be an unrecognized cause of cryptogenic cirrhosis, but it doesn't seem to be the most prevalent.

In France, Duclos-Vallée et al,[12] evaluated 26 patients with cryptogenic cirrhosis from a series of 881 who underwent liver transplantation and found a predominance of autoimmune hepatitis, 14 cases (54%), while NAFLD accounted for 3 cases (11.5%). Of the 3 cases of NAFLD, 2 had NASH and 1 had a recurrence of the disease. Of the 6 cases that remained undiagnosed, none developed hepatitis.

In Germany, in 2009, Heringlake and colleagues[14] found similar results when they retrospectively studied the clinical parameters and histopathology of 126 patients with cryptogenic cirrhosis. The authors found 43 patients who met criteria for autoimmune hepatitis, 22 for NASH, 19 for drug-induced liver injury and 42 remained without an etiological diagnosis. In 20 of the NASH cases, DM, obesity/overweight, dyslipidemia and/or systemic arterial hypertension were found.

It is difficult to prove a causal link between NASH and cryptogenic cirrhosis, since there is a progressive loss of the typical histological findings of the disease as it progresses to cirrhosis.[31-33] As we can see from the studies cited, the causal relationship is suggested by the study of risk factors and/or post-transplant follow-up with liver biopsy.

In order to understand the risk factors and histological findings of NASH, it is necessary to take a brief look at the subject.

NON-ALCOHOLIC STEATOHEPATITIS

NAFLD is defined as the accumulation of fat in the liver exceeding 5 to 10% of its weight.[34] This term was suggested in 1986 by Schaffner and Thaler,[35] to designate this entity whose spectrum varies from steatosis, an apparently benign condition, to steatohepatitis, which can present with liver fibrosis, culminating in cirrhosis in around 22% of patients. , ,[31,32,36,37]

The term non-alcoholic steatohepatitis appeared previously, in 1980, in an article by Ludwig et al.[38] The term was proposed to designate liver biopsy findings similar to alcoholic liver disease in patients with no history of alcohol consumption, surgical *bypass* or use of drugs capable of inducing steatohepatitis.

From a histological point of view, it is necessary to use a staging system that includes a set of findings in order to classify NAFLD across its entire spectrum. The classic histopathological classification was proposed by Brunt and collaborators[39] in 1999. In this study, which focuses on NASH, a grading scheme for necroinflammatory activity and fibrosis staging was proposed. The degree of activity is classified as 1 - mild, 2 - moderate and 3 - intense, and is inferred by a combination of the findings of steatosis with lobular and/or portal inflammation and hepatocellular injury (hepatocyte ballooning). The fibrosis stage ranges from 0 to 4, taking into account the absence (stage 0) or presence of fibrosis: perisinusoidal / pericellular involving Rappaport zone 3 - stage 1; the previous one plus periportal fibrosis - stage 2; the previous two plus bridging fibrosis - stage 3; and cirrhosis - stage 4.[39] These characteristics differentiate it from "simple" steatosis, which presents as fat deposits (triglycerides or phospholipids) in more than 5% of hepatocytes, without necroinflammatory activity or fibrosis.[40]

In 2005, the *NASH Clinical Research Network* developed and validated a histological assessment system that covers the entire spectrum of *NAFLD* and is also valid for pediatric patients, known as the *NAS - NAFLD Activity Score.*[41] This system was based on the classification by Brunt et al.[39] and refined from there, becoming more detailed. A major advantage is that it is useful for measuring histological changes after therapeutic interventions.[41]

The natural history of NAFLD has been investigated by cohort studies, some of which have used serial liver biopsies to assess the evolution of fibrosis.

In 1995, Teli et al.[36] published a study of 40 patients with no history of alcoholism, whose liver biopsy showed the presence of hepatic steatosis only, excluding fibrosis or any other findings suggestive of steatohepatitis. Of the 26 patients alive at the end of follow-up, 14 did not have a repeat biopsy because their ultrasound and aminotransferase levels were normal. Of the 12 cases in which the biopsy was repeated between 7.6 and 16 years later, none had developed cirrhosis or signs of steatohepatitis. Only one case (8.3%) showed progression to fibrosis, thus demonstrating the stable, relatively benign or non-progressive nature of "pure" non-alcoholic steatohepatitis. The authors also compare these data with those found by themselves the previous year, regarding the histological evolution of cases of "pure" alcohol-induced steatosis in patients who continued to drink, when 8 out of 27 (29.6%) patients developed cirrhosis.[42]

Steatohepatitis, in turn, has the potential to evolve into cirrhosis, as has already been demonstrated by some studies in which serial liver biopsies were carried out in a small number of cases.

In 1989, Lee[43] published a study in which he evaluated 49 patients with NASH, 13 of whom underwent serial biopsies. Eight patients remained stable, but the degree of fibrosis progressed in 5 cases (38.4%) and 2 patients developed cirrhosis (15.3%).

The following year, Powell et al.[31] published a study in which they evaluated 42 patients with NASH proven by liver biopsy, carrying out serial biopsies in 13 cases, between 1 and 9 years after the index biopsy. Of the 13 cases, 4 showed histological worsening (30.7%). There was progression from fibrosis to cirrhosis in 1 case and 3 patients who only presented with steatosis and inflammation presented with fibrosis during follow-up.

In the same line of research, a study involving a large number of patients was published in 2005 by Adams et al.[32] 103 patients were evaluated, 50 of whom were being treated with clofibrate or ursodeoxycholic acid. Histology was classified according to the Brunt criteria.[39] Ninety-six patients met the criteria for NASH. The time interval between the first and last biopsies ranged from 0.7 to 21 years, with a median of 3.2 ± 3 years. The results of the study showed that in around a third of the cases, NASH remained stable (34%), in just over a third there was progression of the degree of fibrosis (37%) and in the remainder fibrosis regressed over time (29%). It should be noted that, when looking only at the patients biopsied after 4 years, two thirds (67%) showed fibrosis progression. Of the total, 9 patients progressed to cirrhosis, and in 2 cases there was no fibrosis in the initial biopsy (one after 9 and the other after 15 years). As for the use of clofibrate or ursodeoxycholic acid in almost half of the cases, the authors argue that the drugs did not interfere with the histological course, based mainly on the analysis of their own data, where no statistical difference was found in the course of fibrosis between patients participating in clinical trials and those biopsied for clinical reasons. It is worth noting that the authors found no association between clinical and biochemical variables with the outcome of the evolution of the degree of fibrosis. However, in relation to the speed of fibrosis progression, BMI and the presence of DM proved to be strong independent predictors, as did the initial degree of fibrosis. It is also worth noting that there was no association between the HOMA-IR index and the rate of fibrosis progression.

Also as part of the natural history of the disease, it is worth mentioning the occurrence of HCC. In 2010, Ascha et al.[6] compared the prevalence of HCC among patients with NASH and HCV and found a cumulative annual incidence of 2.6% in NASH cirrhotics and 4% in HCV cirrhotics. Currently, NASH appears to be a less prevalent cause of HCC than other chronic liver diseases, but it is rational to conclude that the occurrence tends to increase as the prevalence of NASH increases.

Some of the cases in the aforementioned studies have shown that, when cirrhosis develops, there is a gradual loss of the histological findings characteristic of NASH.[3] [1,3][2] Due to this peculiarity, it is difficult to attribute the etiology of cirrhosis to NASH when the previous history is unknown. The mechanisms involved in this process are still unclear, but the role of the portosystemic *shunt*, capillarization of the sinusoids, and the possible natural selection of mitochondria less susceptible to oxidative stress are recognized.[11] The portosystemic *shunt* could be responsible for sparing some areas of the liver from fat deposition, as Matsui et al. proved in 1995.[44] The capillarization of the sinusoids, in turn, hinders the passage of large molecules, such as lipoproteins, from the portal circulation to the interior of the hepatocyte.[45] It is known that mitochondrial dysfunction plays a key role in the genesis of steatohepatitis, generating free oxygen radicals and favoring new lesions caused by these same radicals, in a vicious cycle.[46] Due to the genetic polymorphism of mitochondrial DNA, some mitochondria would be more resistant to the action of free radicals, being naturally selected after a period of exposure to oxidative stress. The end result would be a hepatocyte with resistant mitochondria, without much potential for progression from simple steatosis to inflammation and fibrosis.[46]

In the majority of cases, the clinical presentation of NAFLD and steatohepatitis is asymptomatic; occasionally there is fatigue or discomfort in the right hypochondrium. ,[4047] Patients are usually investigated for alterations in aminotransferases, hepatomegaly seen on physical examination or the finding of fatty infiltration detected on ultrasound, but a definitive diagnosis can only be made after liver biopsy and the exclusion of other causes.[40]

With its silent nature, the exact prevalence of NAFLD is unknown.[48] However, it is estimated to be around 20 to 30%, ,[4950] being one of the most common liver diseases. , ,[234951] The prevalence of NASH in the adult population is estimated to be around 3 to 6%,[52] however, an American study[53] carried out in 2011 suggested that this prevalence is even higher, at around 12%. Zamin Jr and collaborators,[54] in a population-based study carried out in Porto Alegre, RS, observed a prevalence of NASH of 3.18% in obese individuals without associated DM. When looking at specific populations of obese or type 2 diabetics, the prevalence of NAFLD rises to up to 70 and 75% respectively,[55] reflecting the association with metabolic syndrome.

The etiology of NAFLD is multivariate. A number of conditions cause triglyceride accumulation in hepatocytes, generating predominantly macrovesicular steatosis, such as: insulin resistance, malnutrition, total parenteral nutrition, use of amiodarone, tamoxifen, methotrexate and corticosteroids. Other situations lead to inhibition of mitochondrial lipid ^-oxidation, causing predominantly microvesicular steatosis, for example: steatohepatitis of pregnancy, use of aspirin, tetracycline, cocaine and exposure to some petrochemicals.[56]

Obesity, particularly central obesity, is one of the conditions that promotes insulin resistance.[57-59] Due to the worldwide obesity "epidemic"[60-63] observed in recent years, insulin resistance can be considered one of the most prevalent causes of NAFLD. The association is so frequent that Pascale et al. advocate abandoning the epithet "non-alcoholic" and introducing the term metabolic steatohepatitis or metabolic fatty liver disease.[64]

Currently, NAFLD is being considered as the hepatic component of metabolic syndrome. ,[5065] This syndrome is a set of risk factors for atherosclerotic cardiovascular disease and brings together conditions that directly promote atherogenesis and insulin resistance. Polycystic ovary syndrome, NAFLD and sleep apnea are examples of entities known to be associated with metabolic syndrome. [66]

According to the consensus led by the *International Diabetes Federation,*[67] published in 2009, the definition of metabolic syndrome must include at least 3 of the following 5 criteria:

- TG>150 mg/dL.

- HDL <40 mg/dL for men and <50 mg/dL for women.

- Systolic blood pressure >130 mmHg and/or diastolic >85 mmHg.

- Fasting glucose >100 mg/dL.

- Abdominal circumference >90 cm in men and >80 cm in women in South America.

This abdominal circumference cut-off point has been modified over time in order to adapt it to the population/racial characteristics of each continent. According to the *American Heart Association* criteria,[66] *in* 2005, the abdominal circumference limit was universal, 102 cm for men and 88 cm for women. This parameter was in the criteria for metabolic syndrome defined by ATP III,[68] in 2001, which in turn removed it from the 1998 American *guideline on* overweight and obesity.[69] The 2009 consensus67 suggests that each country should set its own abdominal circumference limit.

Since the introduction of the two-hit theory by Day and James,[70] in 1998, to explain the pathogenesis of steatosis and its progression to inflammation, fibrosis and cirrhosis, other evidence has been added suggesting the decisive role of insulin resistance in the evolutionary transformation of NAFLD.[71]

The first trigger is the development of steatosis. This process, usually triggered by insulin resistance, occurs due to alterations in lipid metabolism, favoring the accumulation of TG in hepatocytes.[72] In this phase, the role of inhibition of mitochondrial lipid ^-oxidation is also notable, which may be the initial mechanism of NAFLD secondary to drugs.[70]

For hepatic steatosis to progress to inflammation and fibrosis, a second trigger is needed: oxidative stress, which comes from a secondary stimulus, mainly adipocytokines and oxygen free radicals from the mitochondrial respiratory chain.[70,72] The consequence of oxidative stress is lipid peroxidation in the mitochondrial and hepatocyte membrane, leading to the secretion of pro-inflammatory cytokines and activation of stellate cells, resulting in fibrosis.[70,72]

Based on the pathophysiology, some drugs have been studied for the treatment of NASH, but no single therapy has been approved for treatment at the time of this study.[73,74]

Physical exercise and a reduced-calorie diet remain the cornerstones of treatment for NAFLD and NASH, since the loss of adipose tissue reduces insulin resistance.[73] In 2010, Promrat and colleagues[75] carried out a one-year randomized controlled trial to detect the effect of intensive lifestyle intervention on aminotransferase levels and histological findings in NASH. The authors concluded that the magnitude of weight loss correlates strongly with improvement in NASH markers, and that a minimum of 7% weight loss is required to achieve regression in *NAS*. It should be noted that no participant showed an improvement in the degree of fibrosis.

As for bariatric surgery, it is not yet possible to establish its role in the treatment of NAFLD due to the lack of adequate randomized clinical trials, according to a review carried out by the Cochrane database.[76]

Thiazolidinediones are drugs used in the treatment of DM because they improve insulin sensitivity in adipose, hepatic and musculoskeletal tissue.[72] Rosiglitazone and pioglitazone stand out in the literature in the context of NAFLD, but only the latter is currently available.

Neuschwander-Tetri and colleagues[77] carried out a study in which 30 patients with biopsy-proven NASH received 4 mg of rosiglitazone twice a day for 48 weeks. In the 25 patients who completed the study, there was histological improvement in fibrosis and hepatocellular injury, a decrease in aminotransferases and an improvement in insulin sensitivity.

Ratziu et al.[78] conducted a similar randomized study using a control group, and found an improvement in aminotransferase levels and steatosis, with a reduction in insulin resistance, but no improvement in liver fibrosis. As adverse effects, they found a slight reduction in hemoglobin levels, weight gain and painful lower limb edema.

Rosiglitazone, however, appears to be associated with an increased risk of acute myocardial infarction (AMI) and heart failure. In a meta-analysis that included 42 clinical trials of rosiglitazone in the treatment of patients with DM, Nissen and Wolski[79] found an odds ratio for AMI of 1.43 (CI = 1.03 - 1.98). Following this meta-analysis, Home et al. published[80] an interim analysis of the RECORD study, led by the pharmaceutical industry, which showed a higher risk of heart failure in the rosiglitazone group, but found no statistically significant difference between the two groups when analyzing the AMI event, although this data cannot be conclusive. In 2009, the final RECORD report[81] was published, showing an annual rate of around 0.5% of AMIs in the rosiglitazone group. However, Nissen, in a statement published in JAMA[82] in March/2010, calls this data into question.

Pioglitazone has also been evaluated. A pilot study was published in 2004 by Promrat and colleagues[83] evaluating the effects of this drug in 18 non-diabetic patients. The trial was carried out with 30 mg/day of pioglitazone for 48 weeks. At the end of the study, the authors observed histological improvement in two-thirds of cases, a reduction in liver fat content (assessed by magnetic resonance imaging), a drop in alanine aminotransferase levels in 72% of cases, a reduction in fasting insulin by 21% from baseline and in free fatty acids by 16%.

A randomized controlled clinical trial conducted by Belfort et al[84] evaluated the use of 45 mg/day of pioglitazone and a low-calorie diet in 26 patients with DM and NASH (proven by biopsy) versus a control group of 21 similar patients treated with placebo and a low-calorie diet for 6 months. They reported an improvement in glycemic control, aminotransferase levels and hepatic sensitivity to insulin; a reduction in the fat content of the liver (measured by nuclear magnetic resonance); a reduction in necroinflammatory findings, but no significant improvement in fibrosis.

In 2010, the PIVENS study was published,[85] conducted by the *NASH Clinical Research Network,* which compared the effect of 30 mg/day of pioglitazone and 800 IU/day of vitamin E, an antioxidant, with placebo in the treatment of NASH in non-diabetic adults. The study lasted 2 years and liver biopsies were taken before and after the treatment period. Both drugs showed a reduction in *NAS of* 1.9 points versus -0.5 points for placebo, with p <0.001. NASH resolution occurred in 21% of patients taking placebo, 36% of those taking vitamin E (p =0.05) and 47% of those taking pioglitazone (p =0.001). In both treatment groups there was a significant reduction in steatosis, lobular inflammation, aminotransferases, y-glutamyltranspeptidase and alkaline phosphatase when compared to placebo. Ballooning was reduced to a greater extent in both treatment groups, but in the pioglitazone group it only showed a significant difference in a second analysis, removing patients without ballooning in the initial biopsy. None of the drugs showed an improvement in the fibrosis index.

Lutchman et al.[86] evaluated the effect of discontinuing treatment with 30 mg/day of pioglitazone for 1 year in 13 patients with biopsy-proven NASH. They concluded that discontinuation of the drug was associated with increased aminotransferases, decreased adiponectin, decreased insulin sensitivity and increased hepatic fat content.

Other antioxidants, such as betaine, and anti-TNFa, such as pentoxifylline, need further studies to define their therapeutic potential in NASH.[73],[87]

Some studies with metformin, a drug that promotes improved insulin sensitivity, have been carried out in patients with NASH, showing biochemical improvement,[73] but controlled studies are needed to assess histological response.

Genfibrozil, a drug that acts on hypertriglyceridemia, was evaluated in a controlled study that observed an improvement in liver enzymes and TG levels in the treatment group.[88] A pilot study for the treatment of NASH with fenofibrate, published in 2008, showed a biochemical response, but not a histological one.[89]

Ursodeoxycholic acid, a natural component of bile, showed no difference in terms of histological or biochemical improvement compared to placebo in the treatment of NASH.[90]

As you can see, NASH is a disease that has only been characterized for a short period of time, but which has the potential to evolve into cirrhosis. Once cirrhosis has set in, the evolution of these cases is very similar to that of cirrhosis from other causes, with a few but interesting differences that are worth noting.

In 2006, an important prospective study of the natural history of NASH cirrhosis was published,[91] with more than 10 years of cohort follow-up. In this study, the clinical data and evolution of 152 patients with NASH cirrhosis were compared with those of 150 patients with HCV cirrhosis. The cases and controls were very similar in terms of demographic and laboratory profile; the only differences were in the presence of DM, hypercholesterolemia and hypertriglyceridemia, which were more prevalent in the NASH cirrhosis group. The authors observed the development of 10 cases of HCC in 149 patients in the NASH cirrhosis group versus 25 in 147 in the HCV cirrhosis group (p =0.01). It should be noted that cases of cryptogenic cirrhosis, which could represent a more advanced stage of NASH cirrhosis, were excluded. Ascites remained the most common complication; however, patients with NASH cirrhosis had a lower risk of developing ascites compared to controls. Mortality in those with compensated cirrhosis was lower in the NASH cirrhosis group (4% versus 20% of controls), and was similar when decompensated cirrhosis was observed. An interesting and significant difference was the higher mortality from heart disease in NASH cirrhosis cases (8 out of 29) compared to controls (1 out of 44), reflecting the higher prevalence of risk factors for coronary heart disease / congestive heart failure and endothelial dysfunction associated with steatosis.[92]

Despite the difficulty in attributing the etiology of cryptogenic cirrhosis to a case of NASH that has lost its histological features, the effort is justified by the social impact of the disease. As has been said, the prevalence of NASH, although uncertain, accompanies the "epidemic" of obesity that has been observed in recent decades. ,[50][60-63] Given the importance of preventing or treating liver diseases with the potential to develop into cirrhosis, it is essential to investigate whether there is a link between NASH and cryptogenic cirrhosis in our country.

CHAPTER 2 - OBJECTIVES

2.1 General Objective

The validates the possible etiological relationship between non-alcoholic steatohepatitis and cryptogenic cirrhosis.

2.2 Specific objectives

> To determine the prevalence of risk factors for NASH - presence of altered fasting glucose and/or DM, obesity, high total cholesterol (TC) levels, low HDL levels and hypertriglyceridemia - in patients classified as having cryptogenic cirrhosis.

> Compare this prevalence with that of patients diagnosed with NASH and with that of a control group made up of cirrhotics due to alcohol and hepatitis C.

CHAPTER 3 - PATIENTS AND METHODS

3.1 DELINEATION

This was a cross-sectional analytical descriptive study carried out at the Irmandade Santa Casa de Misericórdia de Porto Alegre (ISCMPA) between February 2008 and December 2009, after the research protocol had been analyzed and approved by the hospital's Research Ethics Committee.

3.2 POPULATION

- Inclusion criteria

Patients over the age of 18, being followed up at ISCMPA, classified with one of the diagnoses below, according to the criteria set out below:

(1) NASH - according to clinical assessment and histopathological analysis, according to the Brunt classification.[39] Cirrhotic patients were not included.

(2) Liver cirrhosis - defined by histopathological analysis or by a combination of clinical / laboratory, echographic and endoscopic data (gastro-esophageal varices).

Among the patients who met the criteria for cirrhosis, only those with underlying chronic liver disease were included in the study:

(2.1) Hepatitis C - a positive test for anti-HCV by the 3[a] generation ELISA method is accepted for this diagnosis.

(2.2) Alcohol - according to clinical history of consumption of >40g/day for men for more than 10 years and >20g/day for women for more than 8 years.

(2.3) Cryptogenic - when previous investigation for currently known liver diseases was negative. To this end, the medical records contained a negative history of alcohol consumption, hepatotoxic drugs capable of inducing chronic hepatopathy or occupational exposure to hepatotoxins and tests that refuted the presence of other chronic hepatopathies:

> Viral hepatitis - HBsAg negative, anti-HCV negative.

> Autoimmune hepatitis or CBP - FAN negative, anti-smooth muscle antibody negative, anti-mitochondria antibody negative;

> Metabolic diseases - ceruloplasmin and urinary copper within the normal range to rule out Wilson's disease, normal al-antitrypsin dosage to rule out cirrhosis due to al-antitrypsin deficiency and ferritin dosage <500pg/dL and transferrin saturation index <50% to rule out hemochromatosis.

- Exclusion criteria

Patients whose diagnoses were not fully defined, with most of the data missing from the medical records, with secondary causes of NASH or other causes of cirrhosis such as hepatitis B, autoimmune hepatitis, CBP and hemochromatosis.

3.3 SAMPLE AND PROTOCOL

Cirrhotic patients were enrolled at the ISCMPA Hepatology outpatient clinic and all consecutive patients who met the inclusion criteria were selected. In some cases, not all the data was complete, so when certain variables were analyzed, the number of patients analyzed was lower than the total number of patients allocated to the group.

The medical records sent to the weekly Hepatology outpatient clinic were reviewed to identify the patients who met the inclusion criteria. Those patients who were suitable for the study and came in for a routine consultation were first assessed by the attending doctor for their clinical evolution and to request routine complementary tests. In a second stage, they were approached by the researcher to fill in the Informed Consent Form (Appendix A) and complete the questionnaire (Appendix B). Data obtained by reviewing the medical records of patients identified in the discharge report file of ISCMPA's Gastroenterology and Hepatology Service was also included.

Data collection, based on the questionnaire in Appendix B, was aimed at investigating the main risk factors for primary NASH, which are some of the constituents of metabolic syndrome: low HDL levels, hypertriglyceridemia, presence of altered fasting glucose or DM and obesity, as well as hypercholesterolemia. The HDL value considered low was <40 mg/dL for men and <50 mg/dL for women, while hypertriglyceridemia was considered to be TG >150 mg/dL, according to the criteria for metabolic syndrome.[67] The DM diagnostic criterion adopted is that established by the Brazilian Society of Endocrinology and Metabology, i.e. fasting glycemia >126 mg/dL on two occasions or glycemia >200 mg/dL after 2 hours of overload with 75 g of glucose.[93] Altered fasting glucose is defined as glucose >100 mg/dL, according to the same source. Obesity was defined as BMI (calculated using the formula: weight in kilograms/height in meters^2) >30 kg/m^2 and overweight as BMI between 25 and 29.9kg/m^2 .[94] Hypercholesterolemia was defined as TC >200 mg/dL.[68] Other variables were also assessed to determine the clinical profile of the study groups. Gender, age and severity of liver disease according to the Child-Pugh criteria were recorded.[95] Some tests needed to rule out possible causes of cirrhosis were also recorded in the protocol, as well as a survey on alcohol intake, useful in defining cryptogenic cirrhosis.

The selection of patients with NASH began with a search in the Pathology department at ISCMPA, looking for patients by the histopathology results of liver biopsies diagnosed with steatohepatitis. The medical records were then reviewed to ensure that NASH was clinically and histopathologically correlated. Patients with secondary causes of NASH or alcoholic steatohepatitis were eliminated. No patients were biopsied for the purposes of this study. The age considered was that of the patient at the time of the biopsy, as well as the results of the tests available in the medical records.

The patients were allocated into groups according to their underlying liver disease:

Group 1. NASH

Group 2. Cryptogenic cirrhosis

$$\text{Grupo 3} \begin{cases} \text{Cirrose por álcool} \\ \text{Cirrose por HCV} \\ \text{Cirrose por álcool + HCV} \end{cases}$$

3.4 RESEARCH ETHICS COMMITTEE

The research project for this study was submitted to the Ethics in Research Committee.

ISCMPA Research under protocol number 2045/08, having been approved under opinion number 565/08.

3.5 STATISTICAL ANALYSIS

The data was processed and analyzed using the program

Software: PASW (Predictive Analytical Software for Windows) version 17.

Patients with alcohol cirrhosis, HCV cirrhosis and alcohol cirrhosis associated with HCV were grouped together (group 3) for calculation purposes. Measures of association were made using the prevalence of risk factors for NASH, comparing groups 1 versus 2 and 2 versus 3.

The chi-square test and Fisher's exact test were used for categorical variables and the t-test for continuous variables. Tukey's test was used to compare the means for age, which allows us to determine whether two means are statistically different. Given the design of two primary comparisons, we used the Bonferroni correction to determine statistical significance. This method is used to guarantee the desired level of significance (a) for the group (in this case, a = 0.05) when multiple analyses are carried out, because when more than one analysis is carried out, the chance of a type 1 error increases. Applying the correction is simple: the a of each individual test is adjusted by dividing the desired value of a for the group by the number of comparisons to be made. Therefore, in this study, p-values <0.025 (0.05/2) were considered significant.

CHAPTER 4 - RESULTS

Of the 466 medical records reviewed, 176 were excluded due to the absence of various data, inconclusive diagnosis or secondary cause of NASH. A total of 290 cases were included which contained most of the data to be collected and met the inclusion criteria, allocated into groups as follows:

Group 1. ....NASH47patients

Group 2. Cryptogenic cirrhosis47patients

Grupo 3 { Cirrose por álcool … … … … … … … … … … … … … ….75pacientes / Cirrose por HCV … … … … … … … … … … … … … ….70pacientes } 196 pacientes / Cirrose por álcool + HCV … … … … … … … … …51 pacientes

<u>GENDER</u>

The group with cryptogenic cirrhosis showed a balanced distribution of patients between genders, with 23 females and 24 males. Those with NASH were predominantly female (68.1%). In those cirrhotic due to alcohol and/or HCV, males predominated (64.8%).

The group with cryptogenic cirrhosis is statistically similar to the group with NASH (p = 0.06) and the group with cirrhosis due to alcohol and/or HCV (p = 0.081). Table 1.

Table 1 - Distribution of patients according to gender.

Group	n	Female	Male	p group1 x 2	p group 2 x 3
1. NASH	47	32 (68,1%)	15 (31,9%)	0,06	
2. Cryptogenic C.	47	23 (48,9%)	24 (51,1%)		
3. C. alcohol | HCV	196	69 (35,2%)	127 (64,8%)		0,081

<u>AGE</u>

The mean age of patients with cryptogenic cirrhosis was 52 years, while that of patients with NASH was 46.4 years, around 6 years lower, with a p-value <0.05, which, due to the Bonferroni correction, is not significant. The two cirrhotic groups were similar in terms of mean age. Table 2.

Table 2 - Distribution of patients according to mean age.

Group	n	Average age±SD		p group 1 x 2	p group 2 x 3
1. NASH	47	46,4	± 11,4	0,041	
2. Cryptogenic C.	47	52,0	± 15,8		
3. C. alcohol | HCV	196	53,8	± 9,6		0,570

<u>CHILD-PUGH CLASSIFICATION</u>

The groups of cirrhotic patients were homogeneous in terms of liver disease severity. Table 3.

Table 3 - Distribution of cirrhotic patients according to Child-Pugh criteria.

Group	Child A n		Child B n		Child C n	
2. Cryptogenic C.	28	(59,6%)	14	(29,8%)	05	(10,6%)
3. C. alcohol | HCV	83	(43,5%)	76	(39,8%)	32	(16,8%)

p-value =0.235.

<u>GLICEMIA</u>

The prevalence of altered fasting glucose / DM in patients with cryptogenic cirrhosis was 68.2%. This prevalence was very close to that of patients with NASH, which was 62.8%, being statistically similar, p =0.59.

Comparing the prevalence of altered fasting glucose / DM in the cryptogenic cirrhosis group with that in the alcohol and/or HCV group (45.2%), there was a statistical difference, p =0.006. Table

Table 4 - Distribution of patients according to blood glucose level.

Group	n	mg/dL		p group 1 x 2	p group 2 x 3
		< 100 n	> 100 mg/dL n		
1. NASH	43	16 (37,2%)	27 (62,8%)	0,597	
2. Cryptogenic C.	44	14 (31,8%)	30 (68,2%)		
3. C. alcohol | HCV	188	103 (54,8%)	85 (45,2%)		0,006

<u>BMI</u>

A prevalence of 27.5% obesity and 47.5% overweight was found in patients with cryptogenic cirrhosis, so that 75% of patients were over the ideal weight.

In the NASH group, this figure was 73.8% obesity and 21.4% overweight, i.e. 95.2% of patients had a BMI >25 kg/m^2 , significantly different from the cryptogenic cirrhosis group, p <0.001. In those cirrhotic due to alcohol and/or HCV, the prevalence of obesity was 21.1% - with 62.2% of cases being overweight + obese. In this sample, the cirrhotic groups were statistically similar (p =0.239). Table 5.

One detail about the NASH group - 31 of the 42 patients have a BMI of 30 kg/m or more^2 :

$$\begin{cases} 8\ (25,8\%) \dots \dots \dots \dots \dots \dots \dots 30 - 34,9\ kg/m^2 \\ 9\ (29\%) \dots \dots \dots \dots \dots \dots \dots 35 - 39,9\ kg/m^2 \\ 4\ (33,3\%) \dots \dots \dots \dots \dots \dots \dots \dots \geq 40\ kg/m^2 \end{cases}$$

Table 5 - Distribution of patients according to BMI category.

Group	n	< 25	25 - 29,9	≥30	p group 1 xp group 2	2 x 3
1. NASH	42	02 (4,8%)	09 (21,4%)	31 (73,8%)	< 0,001	
2. C.cryptogenic	**41**	**10 (25%)**	**19 (47,5%)**	**11 (27,5%)**		
3. C. HCV alcohol	171	70 (37,8%)	76 (41,1%)	39 (21,1%)		0,239

LIPID PROFILE

When analyzing the lipid profile, we found that the majority of patients with cryptogenic cirrhosis had normal serum levels of total cholesterol (72.1%) and triglycerides (83.7%), with low levels of HDL. This same pattern was observed in the alcohol and/or HCV cirrhotic group.

In the group with cryptogenic cirrhosis, the prevalence of hypercholesterolemia was 27.9%. This figure is statistically different from the prevalence of the NASH group (62.5%), p =0.002. The group with cirrhosis due to alcohol and/or HCV had a 13.3% prevalence of hypercholesterolemia, and this difference was statistically significant in relation to the group with cryptogenic cirrhosis (p =0.019). Table 6.

Table 6 - Distribution of patients according to serum TC level.

Group	n	< 200 mg/dL n		≥ 200 mg/dL n		p group 1 x 2	p group 2 x 3
1. NASH	40	15	(37,5%)	25	(62,5%)	0,002	
2. Cryptogenic C	**43**	**31**	**(72,1%)**	**12**	**(27,9%)**		
3. C. alcohol|HCV	181	157	(86,7%)	24	(13,3%)		0,019

As for HDL, the analysis was carried out separately for men and women, as shown in the tables below.

Low HDL was found in 36.4% of men with cryptogenic cirrhosis, which is not significantly different from the prevalence found in NASH (53.8%) or cirrhosis caused by alcohol and/or HCV (40.2%). Table 7.

Table 7 - Distribution of male patients according to serum HDL level.

Group	n	< 40 mg/dL n		≥ 40 mg/dL n	
1. NASH	13	07	(53,8%)	06	(46,2%)
2. Cryptogenic C.	22	**08**	**(36,4%)**	14	**(63,6%)**
3. C. alcohol | HCV	107	43	(40,2%)	64	(59,8%)

Between the 3 groups: $x^2 = 1,111$, where p $= 0,574$.

Among the women, low HDL was found in 81% of those in the cryptogenic cirrhosis group. The prevalence found in the other groups was lower, 50.8% in those cirrhotic due to alcohol and/or HCV (p =0.015) and 32% in those with NASH (p <0.001). Table 8.

Table 8 - Distribution of female patients according to serum HDL level.

Group	n	< 50 mg/dL n	≥ 50 mg/dL n	p group 1 x 2	p group 2 x 3
1. NASH	25	08 (32%)	17 (68%)	<0,001	
2. Cryptogenic C.	21	17 (81%)	04 (19%)		
3. C. alcohol | HCV	63	32 (50,8%)	31 (49,2%)		0,015

As for hypertriglyceridemia, the prevalence in the cryptogenic cirrhosis group was 16.3%, which was significantly different from the prevalence in the NASH group (61.5%; p <0.001) and similar to the other cirrhotic group (9.1%; p =0.168). Table 9.

Table 9 - Distribution of patients according to serum TG level.

Group	n	< 150 mg/dL n	≥150 mg/dL n	p group 1 x 2	p group 2 x 3
1. NASH	39	15 (38,5%)	24 (61,5%)	< 0,001	
2. Cryptogenic C	**43**	**36 (83,7%)**	**07 (16,3%)**		
3. C. alcohol|HCV	176	160 (90,9%)	16 (9,1%)		0,168

CHAPTER 5 - DISCUSSION

Cryptogenic cirrhosis represents the final stage of some occult chronic diseases, with non-alcoholic steatohepatitis being one of the underlying diseases responsible for these cases. , ,[9-12][24][25][27-32] ,Given that the prevalence of NASH accompanies the obesity "epidemic",[60-63] the problem is of public health interest.

NAFLD has been considered the hepatic manifestation of metabolic syndrome[50,65] and some studies looking for an association between cryptogenic cirrhosis and NASH ,[9][24-26] deal with the study of the "metabolic profile" of cirrhotic patients, emphasizing DM and obesity.

In this study, we correlated the prevalence of risk factors for NASH among patients with cryptogenic cirrhosis versus patients with NASH proven by liver biopsy and versus patients cirrhotic due to HCV and/or alcohol.

In January 2011, two articles were published on the epidemiology of DGHNA and NASH, one involving a Western population and the other an Eastern population.

The article by Williams et al,[53] , which covers a population living in the USA, involved 328 abstinent people with no known liver disease who underwent ultrasound. Among these, steatosis was found on imaging in 151 (46%), and 134 underwent liver biopsy, regardless of aminotransferases. According to the results of the histopathological examination, there were 40 patients with NASH, which corresponds to 12.2% of the total or 26.5% of those with steatosis on ultrasound. Considering only the patients with NASH diagnosed by biopsy, the authors found a predominance of male patients (65%), with a mean age of around 55 years, 25% diabetic and 80% obese. Of the patients with "pure" steatosis, the majority were also male (58.9%).

The article by Hashimoto and Tokushige[96] provides an updated review of the epidemiology of NASH in Japan. In this study, the gender distribution of 492 patients with biopsy-proven NASH was demonstrated: up to the age of 50, males predominated, and thereafter females.

In the study by Caldwell et al.[9] there was a prevalence of females (56%) in cases of NASH.

In this series, there was a clear prevalence of females in the NASH group, with 68% of cases, and a mean age of 46 years.

As for cryptogenic cirrhosis, the prevalence of one gender over the other is also unclear in the literature. In 4 articles, the prevalence of females was demonstrated. Caldwell et al,[9] 1999, found a prevalence of 70% female, with a mean age of 63 years. In Janus Ong et al,[30] 2001, 60% of the patients were women, with an average age of 50. Sakugawa et al,[25] in 2003, found 73% female patients among those with cryptogenic cirrhosis, with a mean age of 66 years. Tellez-Avila and colleagues,[26] in 2008, studying risk factors for NASH in patients with cryptogenic cirrhosis, found that 61.9% were women, with a mean age of 57 years.

The studies by Suteja et al,[28] in 2004, and Duclos-Vallée et al,[12] in 2005, found a predominance of males, with 62 and 57% prevalence, respectively.

There are also those who reported a balance between the prevalence of both genders. There are at least 3 articles in this situation: Poonawala et al,[24] 2000, who studied 49 patients with cryptogenic cirrhosis and found 55% female and 45% male patients, with a mean age of 54 years; Ayata et al,[10] in 2002, who found 52% female and 48% male patients; and Sanjeevi et al,[29] 2003, with 53% male and 47% female patients.

Similar to the latter are the data from this series. Here, the patients with cryptogenic cirrhosis were almost equally divided between males and females, with a mean age of 52 years.

In articles dealing with serial biopsies in cases of NAFLD, , ,[313243] it is shown that steatohepatitis can progress to cirrhosis over time, so patients with cirrhosis secondary to NASH are older than their peers without cirrhosis. This progression can happen in less than 10 years, as shown in the article by Adams et al,[32] who observed a patient with NASH evolve from F0 to F4 in 9 years or in the article by Powell et al,[31] where this evolution occurred in 8 years.

In the study presented here, the age difference between patients with NASH and those with cryptogenic cirrhosis was 6 years, in line with the time interval required for the disease to progress.

Analysis of the patients in relation to the Child-Pugh criteria reveals that the groups were homogeneous in terms of the severity of the liver disease, and were therefore suitable for comparison. The exams collected referred to the start of cirrhosis follow-up at the ISCMPA, which is perhaps why the highest proportion of cases were in the Child-Pugh A classification. However, adding up the percentage of Child-Pugh B and C patients, 40.4% were in the cryptogenic cirrhosis group and 56.6% in the alcohol and/or HCV cirrhosis group.

As for the presence of altered fasting glucose or DM, one of the factors most associated with insulin resistance, the present study indicates a prevalence of 68.2% in the group with cryptogenic cirrhosis, a figure similar to that found in the NASH group (p =0.597). This figure is not higher than that described by Caldwell et al.[9] (53%), Poonawala et al.[24] (47%) or Sakugawa et al.[25] and Tellez-Avila et al.[26] (40%), as these authors only considered the prevalence of DM and did not include patients with altered fasting glucose.

In this study, the other cirrhotic patients had a different profile, with a prevalence of 45.2% (p =0.006).

In two articles ,[924] evaluating the presence of risk factors for NAFLD in cryptogenic cirrhosis, both described a higher prevalence of obesity in cryptogenic cirrhosis (47%) than in the control group, always with statistical significance. A third study, by Tellez-Avila et al,[26] with a larger sample, found a prevalence of 16.4%. The difference was statistically significant when the control group was assessed together (8.2% obesity in the controls), but there was no difference when assessed separately. As previously mentioned, the prevalence of overweight showed no statistical difference between the groups. The authors attribute this to malnutrition in cirrhotic patients. The conclusion highlights the use of BMI instead of waist circumference, which may have underestimated the number of cases diagnosed as metabolic syndrome.

In the present study, the prevalence of obesity in cryptogenic cirrhosis was 27.5%, higher than that found by Tellez-Avila et al.[26] The prevalence of overweight was 47.5%, so the overall prevalence of overweight patients in cryptogenic cirrhosis was 75%. In the control group of this study (cirrhotic due to HCV and alcohol), the prevalence was around 20% obese and 40% overweight, with no statistical difference compared to the group with cryptogenic cirrhosis. It is unclear whether the evolution of cirrhosis, with the malnutrition and cachexia characteristic of the progression of the disease,[97] may have influenced the body mass indexes found, reducing the proportion of obese people. It is also not possible to assess the extent to which not pairing the cirrhotic groups by age interfered with the results. The prevalence of obesity in the NASH group was 73.8%, higher than that found in the article by Caldwell et al,[9] , which was 64%. Perhaps this difference is partly due to the methodology used. As the NASH group needed a histopathologically proven diagnosis, and no patients were biopsied for the purpose of this study, the patients in the NASH group suffered a selection bias. As described in the methodology, the sample was selected on the basis of biopsies, a considerable number of which were obtained from patients with more significant and persistent alterations in "liver function tests" or those undergoing bariatric surgery. We believe that this could justify the finding that half of the cases (54.7%) had a BMI >35 kg/m^2 or 33% >40 kg/m^2 . In this sample, possibly due to the selection bias of cases with NASH (almost 55% morbidly obese), the proportion of young people (23%) among the cases of cryptogenic cirrhosis and perhaps the evolution of cirrhosis, the group with cryptogenic cirrhosis did not resemble the patients with NASH.

It is possible that the proportion of cirrhotic patients with more advanced disease (40.4% in group 2 and 56.6% in group 3) contributed to the finding of normal (albeit low) TC values and low HDL values, which is one of the limitations of this study. It is known that the liver plays a central role in lipid homeostasis and that the production of TC and HDL decreases with reduced liver function.[98] This was well demonstrated in the article by Habib et al.[99] which correlated TC and its fractions with albumin, total bilirubin, INR, creatinine and MELD score, and found a strong association between HDL and TC levels and liver function tests, to the point of considering HDL a marker of liver function and, when <30 mg/dL, a predictor of pre-liver transplant mortality.

The studies by Caldwell et al.[9] and Poonawala et al.[24] did not assess the lipid profile of the groups studied. The only article found that correlated metabolic syndrome and cryptogenic cirrhosis by evaluating the lipid profile was by Tellez-Avila et al[26] , although they did not distinguish between

HDL or TG, but analyzed both parameters together. In this article, the authors found a prevalence of dyslipidemia in cryptogenic cirrhosis of 54% versus 6% in the control group, made up of cirrhotic patients with HCV, alcohol and autoimmune hepatitis, (p <0.001), which is maintained when analyzing each control subgroup. The article by Ong et al[30] mentions the mean TG values of cases of cryptogenic cirrhosis with and without NASH, but does not determine the prevalence of hypertriglyceridemia. In the present series, 72% of those with cryptogenic cirrhosis and 86% of those cirrhotic due to alcohol and/or HCV had TC levels <200 mg/dL, and an even higher percentage had TG levels <150 mg/dL. Therefore, hypertriglyceridemia was not found in this sample of cryptogenic cirrhosis, which made it different from the NASH group, in which 61.5% of cases had this variable altered.

As for HDL, there was a difference in the pattern between women and men. Of the women with cryptogenic cirrhosis, 81% had low HDL, as opposed to only half of those with cirrhosis due to alcohol and/or HCV, and this difference was significant (p =0.015). However, this pattern was not repeated in men: around 40% of both cirrhotic groups had low HDL. If we consider the unified sample, we find a total of 25 (out of 43) patients with cryptogenic cirrhosis with low HDL levels. This absolute figure represents 58.1% of the sample. On the other hand, the same calculation gives a prevalence of 44.1% among those cirrhotic due to alcohol and HCV. It is therefore possible to state that this sample of cryptogenic cirrhosis has a high prevalence (almost 60%) of low HDL, even though there is no one to compare it with in the studies in the literature. However, this finding should be reflected upon, since the TC levels in the sample are also low. In relation to NASH, with 32% of women with low HDL, women with cryptogenic cirrhosis have a different profile (p =0.11), with a much higher proportion of low HDL. When analyzing the male gender, the profile is similar (p =0.574).

Systemic arterial hypertension, another parameter of the metabolic syndrome, was not assessed here because cirrhotic patients have hemodynamic changes that lead to a decrease in systemic arterial pressure.[100]

In general, given the data evaluated in this study, from an epidemiological point of view we cannot say that the majority of patients with cryptogenic cirrhosis followed up at the ISCMPA come from the evolution of NASH patients, since not all metabolic syndrome parameters were similar between these two groups of patients and differed significantly from the control group.

However, an inference could be made, since the NASH sample turned out to be a few years younger than the average of those with cryptogenic cirrhosis and the glycemia profile was similar to the NASH group and different from the other cirrhotic patients. From all the studies presented in the introduction, the role of insulin resistance in the pathogenesis of NAFLD and its progression to steatohepatitis is clear. And altered fasting glucose correlates strongly with insulin resistance, as stated in the 2005 consensus on metabolic syndrome.[66] Also in this consensus, the authors note that it is not mandatory for patients with insulin resistance to be clinically obese, but that, in general, they have a central fat distribution. Another limitation of this study was that it didn't assess patients' abdominal circumference, but instead used BMI, following the example of studies published in the literature.[9,2][4-26]

The other parameter that didn't find parity with NASH and cryptogenic cirrhosis in our country was the lipid profile, but this analysis is influenced by the fact that the lipid metabolism of cirrhotic patients is altered[98] and the lack of studies in the literature with which to compare it.

Therefore, the only parameters that were not limited by the study design were gender and glycemia, both of which present results similar to those found in the literature that corroborate the existence of a causal relationship between NASH and cryptogenic cirrhosis.

Due to the limitations already described, and the relevance of the topic, it is clear that more comprehensive studies are needed in terms of population, including cirrhosis of other etiologies in the control group, prospective studies and with a larger sample.

CHAPTER 6 - CONCLUSION

In assessing the possible etiological relationship between non-alcoholic steatohepatitis and cryptogenic cirrhosis, it is not possible to establish a causal relationship with the results obtained. The results of this study only allow us to make an inference, given the concordance of the glycemic profile, and the difference between the mean ages, whose p-value was <0.05, which is in line with the progression of the disease over time.

In patients with cryptogenic cirrhosis, the prevalence found was:

✓ altered fasting glucose levels / DM was 68.2%;
✓ obesity, 27.5%;
✓ hypercholesterolemia, 27.9%
✓ low HDL levels, 58.1%, 81% in women and 36.4% in men;
✓ hypertriglyceridemia, 16.3%.

Comparison of these prevalences with the profile of NASH patients shows statistical similarity only between the glycemic profile and HDL levels in male patients. The comparison with other cirrhotic patients shows a statistical difference only between the glycemic profile, TC and HDL levels in female patients.

CHAPTER 7 - BIBLIOGRAPHICAL REFERENCES

1. Schiano TD, Bodenheimer HC. Complications of Chronic Liver Disease. In: Friedman SL, McQuaid KR, Grendell JH, editors. Current diagnosis and treatment in Gastroenterology. 2nd. ed. Lange Medical Books, McGraw-Hill; 2003. p. 63963.

2. Bosch J, D'Amico G, Garcia-Pagan JC. Portal Hypertension. In: Schiff ER, Sorrell MF, Maddrey WC, editors. Schiff's diseases of the liver. 9th. ed. Philadelphia: Lippincott Williams and Wilkins; 2003. p. 428-85.

3. Ikeda K, Saitoh S, Koida I, et al. A multivariate analysis of risk factors for hepatocellular carcinogenesis: a prospective observation of 795 patients with viral and alcoholic cirrhosis. Hepatology. 1993; 18: 47-53.

4. Lauer GM, Walker BD. Hepatitis C virus infection. N Eng J Med. 2001; 345: 41-51.

5. Sangiovanni A, Del Ninno E, Fasani P, De Fazio C, Ronchi G, Romeo R, et al. Increased survival of cirrhotic patients with a hepatocellular carcinoma detected during surveillance. Gastroenterology. 2004; 126: 1005-14.

6. Ascha MS, Hanouneh IA, Lopez R, Tamimi TA, Feldstein AF, Zein NN. The incidence and risk factors of hepatocellular carcinoma in patients with nonalcoholic steatohepatitis. Hepatology. 2010; 51: 1972-8.

7. Ministry of Health [*homepage*]. Brasília, DF: Transplants - Statistical Data [accessed 06 Apr. 2011]. Available at: www.saude.gov.br.

8. Friedman SL. Hepatic Fibrosis. In: Schiff ER, Sorrell MF, Maddrey WC, editors. Schiff's diseases of the liver. 9th. ed. Philadelphia, Lippincott Williams and Wilkins; 2003. p. 409-27.

9. Caldwell SH, Oelsner DH, Iezzoni JC, Hespenheide EE, Battle EH, Driscoll CJ. Cryptogenic cirrhosis: clinical characterization and risk factors for underlying disease. Hepatology. 1999; 29: 664-69.

10. Ayata G, Gordon FD, Lewis WD, Pomfret E, Pomposelli JJ, Jenkins RL, Khettry U. Cryptogenic cirrhosis: clinicopathologic findings at and after liver transplantation. Hum Pathol. 2002; 33: 1098-104.

11. Caldwell SH, Crespo DM. The spectrum expanded: cryptogenic cirrhosis and the natural history of non-alcoholic fatty liver disease. J Hepatol. 2004; 40: 578-84.

12. Duclos-Vallée JC, Yilmaz F, Johanet C, Roque-Afonso AM, Gigou M, Trichet C, et al. Could post-liver transplantation course be helpful for the diagnosis of so called cryptogenic cirrhosis? Clin Transplant. 2005; 19: 591-99.

13. Maheshwari A, Thuluvath PJ. Cryptogenic cirrhosis and NAFLD: are they related? Am J Gastroenterol. 2006; 101: 664-68.

14. Heringlake S, Schútte A, Flemming P, Schmiegel W, Manns MP, Tillmann HL. Presumed cryptogenic liver disease in Germany: high prevalence of autoantibody-negative autoimmune

hepatitis, low prevalence of NASH, no evidence for occult viral etiology. Z Gastroenterol. 2009; 47: 417- 23.

15.   Saunders JB, Walters JR, Davies AP, Paton A. A twenty year prospective study of cirrhosis. Br Med J. 1981; 282: 263-66.

16.   Hodges JR, Millward-Sadler GH, Barbatis C, Wright R. Heterozygous MZ alpha 1-antitrypsin deficiency in adults with chronic active hepatitis and cryptogenic cirrhosis. N Engl J Med. 1981; 304: 557-60.

17.   Islam N, Khan M, Ahmed Z. Cirrhosis of liver. Bangladesh Med Res Counc Bull. 1981; 7: 45-51.

18.   Keating JJ, Johnson RD, Johnson PJ, Williams R. Clinical course of cirrhosis in young adults and therapeutic potential of liver transplantation. Gut. 1985; 26: 1359-63.

19.   Keating JJ, O'Brien CJ, Stellon AJ, Portmann BC, Johnson RD, Johnson PJ, Williams R. Influence of aetiology, clinical and histological features on survival in chronic active hepatitis: an analysis of 204 patients. Q J Med. 1987; 62: **59-66**.

20.   Tanaka R, Itoshima T, Nagashima H. Follow-up study of 582 liver cirrhosis patients for 26 years in Japan. Liver. 1987; 7: **316-24**.

21.   Olano FC, Romero RP, Pons Mihano JA, Miras López M. Clinical and epidemiological features of hepatic cirrhosis. Analysis of 200 patients. Aten Primaria. 1989; 6: 583-8.

22.   Kodali VP, Gordon SC, Silverman AL, McCray DG. Cryptogenic liver disease in the United States: further evidence for non-A, non-B, non-C hepatitis. Am J Gastroenterol. 1994; 89: 1836-39.

23.   Byron D, Minuk GY. Clinical hepatology: profile of an urban, hospital-based practice. Hepatology. 1996; 24: 813-15.

24.   Poonawala A, Nair SP, Thuluvath PJ. Prevalence of obesity and diabetes in patients with cryptogenic cirrhosis: a case-control study. Hepatology. 2000; 32: 689-92.

25.   Sakugawa H, Nakasone H, Nakayoshi T, Kawakami Y, Yamashiro T, Maeshiro T, et al. Clinical characteristics of patients with cryptogenic liver cirrhosis in Okinawa, Japan. Hepatogastroenterology. 2003; 50: 2005-08.

26.   Tellez-Avila FI, Sanchez-Avila F, García-Saenz-De-Sicilia M, Chavez-Tapia NC, Franco-Guzman AM, Lopez-Arce G, et al. Prevalence of metabolic syndrome, obesity and diabetes type 2 in cryptogenic cirrhosis. World J Gastroenterol. 2008; 14: 4771-75.

27.   Kim WR, Poterucha JJ, Porayko MK, Dickson ER, Steers JL, Wiesner RH. Recurrence of nonalcoholic steatohepatitis following liver transplantation. Transplantation. 1996; 62: 1802-05.

28.   Sutedja DS, Gow PJ, Hubscher SG, Elias E. Revealing the cause of cryptogenic cirrhosis by posttransplant liver biopsy. Transplant Proc. 2004; 36: 2334-37.

29.   Sanjeevi A, Lyden E, Sunderman B, Weseman R, Ashwathnarayan R, Mukherjee S. Outcomes of liver transplantation for cryptogenic cirrhosis: a singlecenter study of 71 patients. Transplant Proc. 2003; 35: 2977-80.

30. Ong J, Younossi ZM, Reddy V, Price LL, Gramlich T, Mayes J, Boparai N. Cryptogenic cirrhosis and posttransplantation nonalcoholic fatty liver disease. Liver Transpl. 2001; 7: 797-801.

31. Powell EE, Cooksley WG, Hanson R, Searle J, Halliday JW, Powell LW. The natural history of nonalcoholic steatohepatitis: a follow-up study of forty-two patients for up to 21 years. Hepatology. 1990; 11: 74-80.

32. Adams LA, Sanderson S, Lindor KD, Angulo P. The histological course of nonalcoholic fatty liver disease: a longitudinal study of 103 patients with sequential liver biopsies. J Hepatol. 2005; 42: 132-8.

33. Clark ME, Ghotb A, Merriman RB. Longitudinal Histologic Evidence of Loss of Steatosis with Progression of NAFLD to Cirrhosis and Liver Transplantation. Gastroenterology. 2009; 136 (Suppl 1): A-847.

34. Cairns SR, Peters TJ. Biochemical analysis of hepatic lipid in alcoholic and diabetic and control subjects. Clin Sci. 1983; 65: 645-52.

35. Schaffner F, Thaler H. Nonalcoholic fatty liver disease. Prog Liver Dis. 1986; 8: 283-98.

36. Teli MR, James OF, Burt AD, Bennett MK, Day CP. The natural history of nonalcoholic fatty liver: a follow-up study. Hepatology. 1995; 22: 1714-19.

37. Matteoni CA, Younossi ZM, Gramlich T, Boparai N, Liu YC, McCullough AJ. Nonalcoholic fatty liver disease: a spectrum of clinical and pathological severity. Gastroenterology. 1999; 116: 1413-19.

38. Ludwig J, Viggiano TR, Mcgill DB, Oh BJ. Nonalcoholic steatohepatitis. Mayo Clinic experiences with a hitherto unnamed disease. Mayo Clin Proc. 1980; 55: 434-8.

39. Brunt EM, Janney CG, Di Bisceglie AM, Neuschwander-Tetri BA, Bacon BR. Nonalcoholic Steatohepatitis: A Proposal for Grading and Staging the Histological Lesions. Am J Gastroenterol. 1999; 94: 2467-74.

40. Mezey E. Fatty Liver. In: Schiff ER, Sorrell MF, Maddrey WC, editors. Schiff's diseases of the liver. 9th. ed. Philadelphia, Lippincott Williams and Wilkins; 2003. p. 1290-304.

41. Kleiner DE, Brunt EM, Van Natta M, Behling C, Contos MJ, Cummings OW, et al. Design and Validation of a Histological Scoring System for Nonalcoholic Fatty Liver Disease. Hepatology. 2005; 41: 1313-21.

42. Teli MR, Day CP, Burt AD, James OF. Pattern of steatosis and continued drinking predict risk of progression to cirrhosis in pure alcoholic fatty liver. Hepatology. 1994; 20: 319A.

43. Lee, RG. Nonalcoholic steatohepatitis: A study of 49 patients. Human Pathology. 1989; 20: 594-8.

44. Matsui O, Kadoya M, Takahashi S, Yoshikawa J, Gabata T, Takashima T, Kitagawa K. Focal sparing of segment IV in fatty livers shown by sonography and CT: correlation with aberrant gastric venous drainage. AJR. 1995; 164: 1137-40.

45. Schaffner F, Popper H. Capillarization of hepatic sinusoids. Gastroenterology. 1963; 44:

239-42.

46.   Begriche K, Igoudjil A, Pessayre D, Fromenty B. Mitochondrial dysfunction in NASH: Causes, consequences and possible means to prevent it. Mitochondrion. 2006; 6: 1-28.

47.   Reid AE. Nonalcoholic Steatohepatitis. Gastroenterology. 2001; 121: 710-23.

48.   American Gastroenterological Association. AGA technical review on nonalcoholic fatty liver disease. Gastroenterology. 2002; 123: 1705-25.

49.   Clark JM, Brancati FL, Diehl AME. Nonalcoholic fatty liver disease: the most common cause of abnormal liver enzymes in the U.S. population. Gastroenterology. 2001; 120: A65.

50.   Farrell GC, Larter CZ. Nonalcoholic fatty liver disease: from steatosis to cirrhosis. Hepatology. 2006; 43: S99-S112.

51.   Daniel S, Ben-Menachem T, Vasudevan G, Ma CK, Blumenkehl M. Prospective evaluation of unexplained chronic liver transaminase abnormalities in asymptomatic and symptomatic patients. Am J Gastroenterol. 1999; 94: 3010 - 14.

52.   Torres DM, Harrison SA. Diagnosis and Therapy of Nonalcoholic Steatohepatitis. Gastroenterology. 2008; 134: 1682-98.

53.   Williams CD, Stengel J, Asike MI, Torres DM, Shaw J, Contreras M, et al. Prevalence of nonalcoholic fatty liver disease and nonalcoholic steatohepatitis among a largely middle-aged population utilizing ultrasound and liver biopsy: a prospective study. Gastroenterology. 2011; 140: 124-31.

54.   Zamin I, Jr, Mattos AA, Zettler CG. Nonalcoholic steatohepatitis in nondiabetic obese patients. Can J Gastroenterol. 2002; 16: 303-7.

55.   Neuschwander-Tetri BA, Caldwell SH. Nonalcoholic Steatohepatitis: Summary of an AASLD single topic conference. Hepatology. 2003; 37: 1202-19.

56.   Loria P, Adinolfi LE, Bellentani S, Bugianesi E, Grieco A, Fargion S, et al. Practice guidelines for the diagnosis and management of nonalcoholic fatty liver disease. A decalogue from the Italian Association for the Study of the Liver (AISF) Expert Committee. Dig Liver Dis. 2010; 42: 272-82.

57.   Jensen MD, Haymond MW, Rizza RA, Cryer PE, Miles JM. Influence of body fat distribution on free fatty acid metabolism in obesity. J Clin Invest. 1989; 83: 1168 - 73.

58.   Abate N, Garg A, Peshock RM, Stray-Gundersen J, Grundy SM. Relationships of generalized and regional adiposity to insulin sensitivity in men. J Clin Invest. 1995; 96: 88 -98.

59.   Raji A, Seely EW, Arky RA, Simonson DC. Body fat distribution and insulin resistance in healthy Asian Indians and Caucasians. J Clin Endocrinol Metab. 2001; 86: 5366 -71.

60.   Mokdad AH, Ford ES, Bowman BA, Dietz WH, Vinicor F, Bales VS, Marks JS. Prevalence of obesity, diabetes, and obesity-related health risk factors, 2001. JAMA. 2003; 289: 76-9.

61.   Sturm R. Increases in clinically severe obesity in the United States, 1986-2000. Arch Intern

Med. 2003; 163: 2146-148.

62. Wang Y, Mi J, Shan XY, Wang QJ, Ge KY. Is China facing an obesity epidemic and the consequences? The trends in obesity and chronic disease in China. Int J Obes. 2007; 31: 177-88.

63. Berghofer A, Pischon T, Reinhold T, Apovian CM, Sharma AM, Willich SN. Obesity prevalence from a European perspective: a systematic review. BMC Public Health. 2008; 8: 200-9.

64. Pascale A, Pais R, Ratziu V. An overview of nonalcoholic steatohepatitis: past, present and future directions. J Gastrointestin Liver Dis. 2010; 19: 415-23.

65. Marchesini G, Brizi M, Bianchi G, Tomassetti S, Bugianesi E, Lenzi M et al. Nonalcoholic fatty liver disease - a feature of the metabolic syndrome. Diabetes. 2001; 50: 1844-50.

66. Grundy SM, Cleeman JI, Daniels SR, Donato KA, Eckel RH, Franklin BA, et al. Diagnosis and Management of the Metabolic Syndrome: an American Heart Association/National Heart, Lung, and Blood Institute Scientific Statement. Circulation. 2005; 112: 2735-52.

67. Alberti KG, Eckel RH, Grundy SM, Zimmet PZ, Cleeman JI, Donato KA, et al. Harmonizing the metabolic syndrome: a joint interim statement of the International Diabetes Federation Task Force on Epidemiology and Prevention; National Heart, Lung, and Blood Institute; American Heart Association; World Heart Federation; International Atherosclerosis Society; and International Association for the Study of Obesity. Circulation. 2009; 120: 1640-45.

68. Executive Summary of The Third Report of The National Cholesterol Education Program (NCEP) Expert Panel on Detection, Evaluation, and Treatment of High Blood Cholesterol in Adults (Adult Treatment Panel III). JAMA. 2001; 285: 2486-97.

69. Clinical guidelines on the identification, evaluation, and treatment of overweight and obesity in adults - the Evidence Report. National Institutes of Health. Obes Res. 1998; 6 (Suppl 2): 51S-209S.

70. Day CP, James OF. Steatohepatitis: a tale of two "hits"? Gastroenterology. 1998; 114: 842-5.

71. Sanyal AJ, Campbell-Sargent C, Mirshahi F, Rizzo WB, Contos MJ, Sterling RK, et al. Nonalcoholic steatohepatitis: association of insulin resistance and mitochondrial abnormalities. Gastroenterology. 2001; 120: 1183-92.

72. Rector RS, Thyfault JP, Wei Y, Ibdah JA. Non-alcoholic fatty liver disease and the metabolic syndrome: an update. World J Gastroenterol. 2008; 14: 185-92.

73. Younossi ZM. Review article: current management of non-alcoholic fatty liver disease and non-alcoholic steatohepatitis. Aliment Pharmacol Ther. 2008; 28: 212.

74. Satapathy SK, Sanyal AJ. Novel treatment modalities for nonalcoholic steatohepatitis. Trends Endocrinol Metab. 2010; 21: 668-75.

75. Promrat K, Kleiner DE, Niemeier HM, Jackvony E, Kearns M, Wands JR, et al. Randomized controlled trial testing the effects of weight loss on nonalcoholic steatohepatitis. Hepatology. 2010; 51: 121-9.

76. Chavez-Tapia NC, Tellez-Avila FI, Barrientos-Gutierrez T, Mendez-Sanchez N, Lizardi-Cervera J, Uribe M. Bariatric surgery for non-alcoholic steatohepatitis in obese patients.

Cochrane Database Syst Rev. 2010; 1: CD007340.

77. Neuschwander-Tetri BA, Brunt EM, Wehmeier KR, Oliver D, Bacon BR. Improved nonalcoholic steatohepatitis after 48 weeks of treatment with the PPAR-gamma ligand rosiglitazone. Hepatology. 2003; 38: 1008-17.

78. RatziuV, Giral P, Jacqueminet S, Charlotte F, Hartemann-Heurtier A, Serfaty L, et al. Rosiglitazone for nonalcoholic steatohepatitis: one-year results of the randomized placebo-controlled fatty liver improvement with rosiglitazone therapy (FLIRT) trial. Gastroenterology. 2008; 135: 100-10.

79. Nissen SE, Wolski K. Effect of Rosiglitazone on the risk of myocardial infarction and death from cardiovascular causes. N Engl J Med. 2007; 356: 2457-71. Erratum in: N Engl J Med. 2007; 357: 100.

80. Home PD, Pocock SJ, Beck-Nielsen H, Gomis R, Hanefeld M, Jones NP, et al. Rosiglitazone evaluated for cardiovascular outcomes - an interim analysis. N Engl J Med. 2007; 357: 28-38.

81. Home, PD, Pocock SJ, Beck-Nielsen H, Curtis PS, Gomis R, Hanefeld M, et al. RECORD Study Team. Rosiglitazone evaluated for cardiovascular outcomes in oral agent combination therapy for type 2 diabetes (RECORD): a multicentre, randomized, open-label trial. Lancet. 2009; 373: 2125-35.

82. Nissen SE. Setting the RECORD Straight. JAMA. 2010; 303: 1194-5.

83. Promrat K, Lutchman G, Uwaifo GI, Freedman RJ, Soza A, Heller T, et al. A pilot study of pioglitazone treatment for nonalcoholic steatohepatitis. Hepatology. 2004; 39: 188-96.

84. Belfort R, Harrison SA, Brown K, Darland C, Finch J, Hardies J, et al. A placebo- controlled trial of pioglitazone in subjects with nonalcoholic steatohepatitis. N Engl J Med. 2006; 355: 2297-307.

85. Sanyal AJ, Chalasani N, Kowdley KV, McCullough A, Diehl AM, Bass NM, et al. Pioglitazone, Vitamin E, or Placebo for Nonalcoholic Steatohepatitis. Engl J Med. 2010; 362: 1675-85.

86. Lutchman G, Modi A, Kleiner DE, Promrat K, Heller T, Ghany M, et al. The effects of discontinuing pioglitazone in patients with nonalcoholic steatohepatitis. Hepatology. 2007; 46: 424-29.

87. Li W, Zheng L, Sheng C, Cheng X, Qing L, Qu S. Systematic review on the treatment of pentoxifylline in patients with non-alcoholic fatty liver disease. Lipids in Health and Disease. 2011; 10: 49-54.

88. Basaranoglu M, Acbay O, Sonsuz A. A controlled trial of gemfibrozil in the treatment of patients with nonalcoholic steatohepatitis.J Hepatol. 1999; 31: 384.

89. Fernández-Miranda C, Pérez-Carreras M, Colina F, López-Alonso G, Vargas C, Solís-Herruzo JA. A pilot trial of fenofibrate for the treatment of non-alcoholic fatty liver disease. Dig Liver Dis. 2008; 40: 200-5.

90. Lindor KD, Kowdley KV, Heathcote EJ, Harrison ME, Jorgensen R, Angulo P, et al.

Ursodeoxycholic acid for treatment of nonalcoholic steatohepatitis: results of a randomized trial. Hepatology. 2004; 39: 770-8.

91. Sanyal AJ, Banas C, Sargeant C, Luketic VA, Sterling RK, Stravitz RT, et al. Similarities and differences in outcomes of cirrhosis due to nonalcoholic steatohepatitis and hepatitis C. Hepatology. 2006; 43: 682-9.

92. Villanova N, Moscatiello S, Ramilli S, Bugianesi E, Magalotti D, Vanni E, et al. Endothelial dysfunction and cardiovascular risk profile in nonalcoholic fatty liver disease. Hepatology. 2005; 42: 473-80.

93. Brazilian Society of Endocrinology and Metabology. Diabetes Mellitus: Classification and Diagnosis. Guidelines Project. Vol 4. Brazilian Medical Association and Federal Council of Medicine. 2004. [Accessed on October 7, 2008]. Available at: www.projetodiretrizes.org.br.

94. Brazilian Society of Endocrinology and Metabology. Obesity: Treatment. Guidelines Project. Vol. 4. Brazilian Medical Association and Federal Council of Medicine. 2006. [Accessed on October 7, 2008]. Available at www.projetodiretrizes.org.br.

95. Pugh RN, Murray-Lyon IM, Dawson JL. Transection of the oesophagus for bleeding oesophageal varices. Br J Surg. 1973; 60: 646-9.

96. Hashimoto E, Tokushige K. Prevalence, gender, ethnic variations, and prognosis of NASH. J Gastroenterol. 2011; 46 (Suppl 1): 63-9.

97. Heitor R. Hepatic Encephalopathy. In: Mattos AA, Dantas-Corrêa EB. Treatise on Hepatology. Rio de Janeiro: Editora Rubio; 2010. p. 523-35.

98. Roy-Chowdhury N, Roy-Chowdhury J. Liver Physiology and Energy Metabolism. In: Feldman M, Friedman LS, Brandt LJ. Sleisenger and Fordtran's Gastrointestinal and Liver Disease: Pathophysiology, Diagnosis, Management. 9th. ed. Philadelphia: Saunders-Elsevier; 2010. p. 1207-25.

99. Habib A, Mihas AA, Abou-Assi SG, Williams LM, Gavis E, Pandak WM, Heuman DM. High-density lipoprotein cholesterol as an indicator of liver function and prognosis in noncholestatic cirrhotics. Clin Gastroenterol Hepatol. 2005; 3: 286-91.

100. Liu H, Gaskari SA, Lee SS. Cardiac and vascular changes in cirrhosis: Pathogenic mechanisms. World J Gastroenterol. 2006; 12: 837-42.

APPENDIX A

INFORMED CONSENT FORM

BROTHERHOOD OF THE HOLY HOUSE OF MERCY OF PORTO ALEGRE

GASTROENTEROLOGY AND HEPATOLOGY SERVICE

RESEARCH TITLE: ETIOLOGICAL ROLE OF
NON-ALCOHOLIC STEATOHEPATITIS
IN CRYPTOGENIC CIRRHOSIS.

We are carrying out a survey with the intention of collecting health data on patients who have cirrhosis of the liver or fatty liver disease. The aim of the study is to compare changes in the health of these patients in terms of cholesterol levels, the presence of diabetes, weight adequacy and liver disease status.

The data obtained will be that contained in the medical records, including your weight and height. You will not have to undergo any extra procedures to take part in the research. Participation in this research does not generate any risk or expense for you, nor will it bring you any immediate private benefit.

Your personal identity will not be exposed in the study.

You are not obliged to take part in the study. And whether or not you take part, you will continue to be monitored for your illness by the medical team at the Santa Casa Hepatology Outpatient Clinic. We are happy to answer any questions you may have. Research Ethics Committee telephone number: (51) 3214-8571.

I, , Record No., authorize the collection of data from my record and the use of the information

obtained for clinical research purposes and subsequent publication in a scientific journal. In view of

the explanations provided, I consider myself to have been informed about the purpose of the study,

the procedure used, the absence of harm and the guarantee of confidentiality regarding the

information provided.

____

Researcher's signature (Andrea Benevides)   *Signature of patient or guardian*

Signature of witness

Porto Alegre,   200_

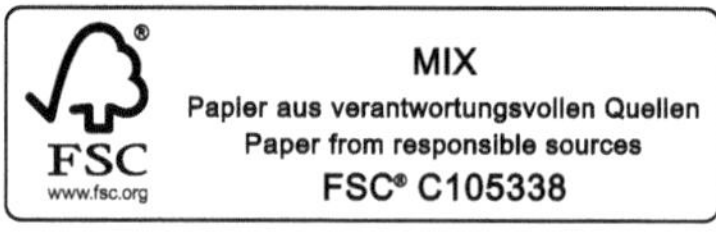

Printed by Books on Demand GmbH, Norderstedt / Germany